Juicing for Cancer

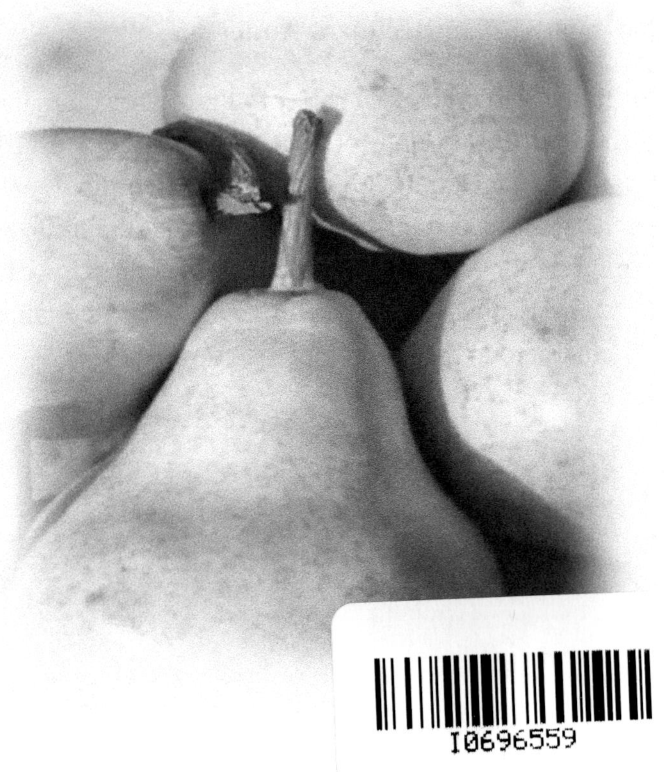

Hector A. Anderson

Table of Contents

Introduction

In this book, we will explore the transformative potential of juicing as a complementary approach to cancer treatment and prevention. Whether you or a loved one is facing a cancer diagnosis or you simply want to adopt a proactive lifestyle to reduce your risk, this book will provide you with valuable insights and practical guidance.

First and foremost, I would like to express my heartfelt appreciation to all the cancer patients, survivors, and their families who have generously shared their personal stories, experiences, and successes with juicing. Your bravery and resilience inspire us all, and it is with your journeys in mind that I have crafted this book.

I would also like to extend my gratitude to the medical professionals, nutritionists, and researchers who have dedicated their careers to the field of oncology and nutritional science. Their expertise and invaluable contributions have shaped the information presented in this book, ensuring that it is based on the latest research and medical knowledge.

The Power of Juicing: Understanding the Benefits for Cancer Patients

Cancer is a complex and multifaceted disease that affects millions of people around the world. It is characterized by the uncontrolled growth and spread of abnormal cells, posing significant challenges to physical and emotional well-being. While medical advancements have improved cancer treatment options, many patients are seeking additional strategies to support their healing journey.

One such approach gaining widespread attention is juicing. Juicing involves extracting the liquid from fruits, vegetables, and herbs, which concentrates their nutritional content into a highly absorbable form. By consuming fresh, nutrient-dense juices, cancer patients can provide their bodies with a potent infusion of vitamins, minerals, antioxidants, and phytochemicals. These bioactive compounds have been found to possess various beneficial properties, including antioxidant, anti-inflammatory, immune-boosting, and detoxifying effects.

Research suggests that juicing can play a role in cancer prevention and treatment by nourishing the body, promoting cellular health, and enhancing the immune system. The high concentration of nutrients in fresh juices can help address nutritional deficiencies commonly experienced by cancer patients due to poor appetite, side effects of treatments, and overall compromised health. Furthermore, the antioxidants found in fruits and vegetables can help neutralize harmful free radicals, reducing oxidative stress and supporting the body's natural defense mechanisms.

Disclaimer and Important Considerations

Before delving into the world of juicing for cancer, it is essential to acknowledge that this book is not a substitute for professional medical advice. The information provided here is meant to complement, not replace, the guidance of qualified healthcare professionals. Every individual's cancer journey is unique, and what works for one person may not be suitable for another.

It is crucial to consult with your healthcare team before making any significant dietary changes, including incorporating juicing into your regimen. They can provide personalized recommendations based on your specific diagnosis, treatment plan, and overall health status. They will consider factors such as any existing dietary restrictions, potential interactions with medications, and the overall nutritional needs of your body.

Additionally, it is important to note that juicing should not be considered a standalone treatment for cancer. It is best utilized as a part of a comprehensive approach that includes medical treatments, proper nutrition, exercise, stress management, and emotional support. Juicing should be viewed as a complementary tool to support overall health and well-being during the cancer journey.

In the following chapters, we will explore the essential ingredients for cancer-fighting juices, design personalized juice protocols, provide delicious recipes, discuss the integration of juicing into cancer treatment plans, and address common questions and concerns. Together, let us embark on this empowering journey of nourishing our bodies and embracing the healing power of juicing in the face of cancer.

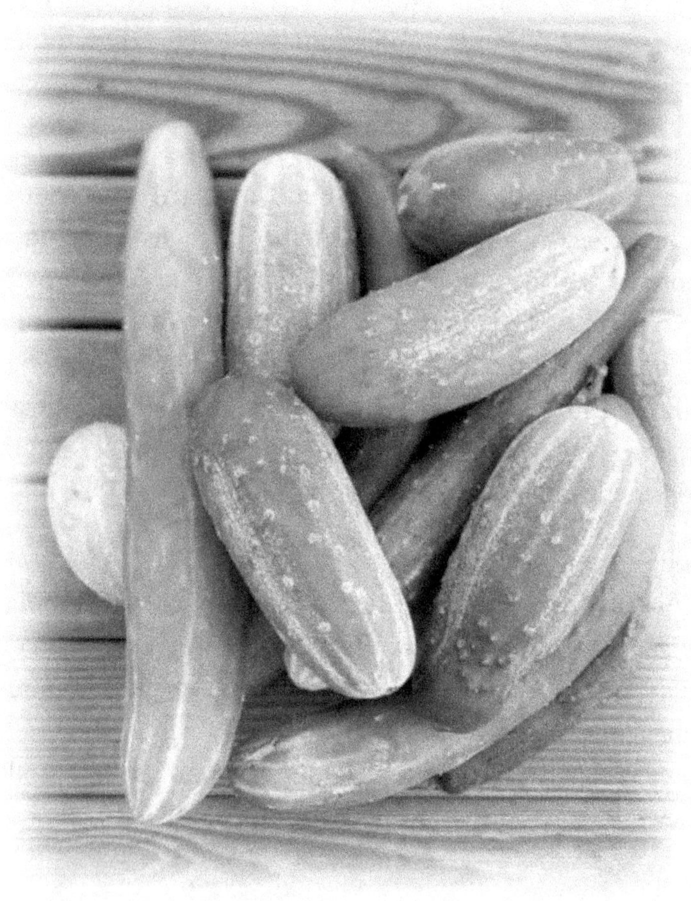

Chapter 1

Understanding Cancer

Cancer is a term used to describe a group of diseases characterized by uncontrolled cell growth and spread. These cells can invade and destroy surrounding tissues, impairing the normal functioning of organs and systems within the body. Cancer can develop in almost any part of the body and may manifest in various forms, each with its own unique characteristics and behaviors.

At its core, cancer occurs when the body's natural processes of cell growth, division, and death are disrupted. Normally, cells grow and divide in an orderly manner to replace damaged or old cells. However, in the case of cancer, genetic mutations or abnormalities occur, leading to uncontrolled cell division and the formation of a mass of cells called a tumor.

Tumors are categorised into two types: benign and malignant. Non-cancerous benign tumors do not infiltrate neighboring tissues or spread to other sections of the body. They can usually be removed through surgical intervention and are less likely to recur. On the other hand, malignant tumors are cancerous and have the ability to invade surrounding tissues and metastasize, spreading to distant organs through the bloodstream or lymphatic system.

Common Types of Cancer and Their Treatment Options

There are numerous types of cancer, each with its own unique characteristics, patterns of growth, and treatment options. Some of the most prevalent forms of cancer include breast cancer, lung cancer, colorectal cancer, prostate cancer, and skin cancer. However, it is important to note that cancer can affect any part of the body and can occur in various organs and systems.

Treatment options for cancer are diverse and depend on several factors, including the type and stage of cancer, the location and size of the tumor, the individual's overall health, and personal preferences. The most often used treatment techniques are surgery, radiation therapy, chemotherapy, immunotherapy, targeted therapy, and hormone therapy. Often, a combination of these approaches is employed to provide the most effective treatment outcome.

The Importance of Nutrition in the Prevention and Treatment of Cancer

Proper nutrition plays a crucial role in cancer prevention and treatment. A balanced diet that is rich in a variety of fruits, vegetables, whole grains, lean proteins, and healthy fats provides the body with essential nutrients, vitamins, minerals, and antioxidants necessary for optimal cellular function and overall well-being. Conversely, a diet that is high in processed foods, unhealthy fats, and added sugars can contribute to chronic inflammation, oxidative stress, and an increased risk of cancer development.

Research has shown that certain dietary factors can influence cancer risk. For instance, diets high in fruits and vegetables have been associated with a lower risk of developing certain types of cancer, such as lung, colorectal, and stomach cancers. These foods are abundant in vitamins, minerals, fiber, and phytochemicals that possess antioxidant and anti-inflammatory properties, helping to protect cells from damage and inhibit the growth of cancer cells.

The Benefits of Juicing for Cancer Patients

Juicing offers a convenient and effective way to incorporate a wide variety of fruits, vegetables, and herbs into the diet, providing concentrated amounts of nutrients in an easily digestible form. For cancer patients, who may experience challenges in consuming adequate amounts of food due to treatment side effects or poor appetite, juicing can be a valuable tool to ensure the body receives essential nutrients.

The benefits of juicing for cancer patients are multi-fold. Firstly, fresh juices provide a rich source of vitamins, minerals, and antioxidants that support immune function, enhance cellular health, and aid in the body's natural detoxification processes. These nutrients help fortify the body's defenses, promote healing, and optimize overall well-being during the cancer journey.

Secondly, juicing can be a gentle way to introduce a variety of plant-based compounds with potential anti-cancer properties into the body. Certain fruits and vegetables, such as berries, cruciferous vegetables, turmeric, ginger, and leafy greens, contain bioactive compounds that have demonstrated anti-inflammatory, antioxidant, and anti-cancer effects in scientific studies.

Additionally, juicing can help alleviate some of the side effects associated with cancer treatments. For example, certain juices may soothe digestive issues, such as nausea or constipation, while others may boost energy levels and combat fatigue.

It is important to note that while juicing can provide valuable nutritional support, it should not be considered a standalone treatment for cancer. Juicing should always be integrated into a comprehensive approach to cancer management, under the guidance of healthcare professionals.

Chapter 2

Exploring the Nutritional Powerhouse: Fruits and Vegetables

Fruits and vegetables are the foundation of a healthy diet and are often referred to as nutritional powerhouses. They are packed with essential vitamins, minerals, fiber, and a wide range of bioactive compounds that contribute to overall health and well-being. When it comes to cancer prevention and treatment, these plant-based foods play a vital role in supporting the body's natural defense mechanisms and promoting optimal cellular function.

Including a diverse array of fruits and vegetables in your juicing regimen can provide a broad spectrum of nutrients that support immune function, reduce inflammation, and provide antioxidant protection. Different fruits and vegetables offer unique profiles of vitamins, minerals, and phytochemicals, so it is important to vary your selection to maximize nutritional benefits.

Crucial Antioxidants and Phytochemicals for Cancer Prevention

Antioxidants and phytochemicals are bioactive compounds found in fruits and vegetables that have been extensively studied for their potential role in cancer prevention. These compounds work by neutralizing harmful free radicals, reducing oxidative stress, and protecting cells from damage.

Some well-known antioxidants include vitamin C, vitamin E, beta-carotene, and selenium. These antioxidants are abundant in fruits and vegetables such as berries, citrus fruits, spinach, kale, carrots, and tomatoes. In addition to their antioxidant properties, they have been associated with a lower risk of certain types of cancer, including lung, breast, prostate, and colorectal cancers.

Phytochemicals are naturally occurring compounds found in plants that provide health benefits beyond basic nutrition. Examples of phytochemicals include flavonoids, carotenoids, and polyphenols. These compounds have been shown to possess anti-inflammatory, anti-cancer, and immune-boosting properties. Some rich sources of phytochemicals include blueberries, cruciferous vegetables (such as broccoli and cauliflower), green tea, turmeric, and garlic.

Superfoods for Enhancing Immunity and Detoxification

Certain foods have gained recognition as "superfoods" due to their exceptional nutritional profiles and potential health benefits. These superfoods can be excellent additions to cancer-fighting juices, as they provide concentrated amounts of nutrients that support immunity and detoxification processes in the body.

Examples of superfoods for enhancing immunity include berries (such as blueberries, strawberries, and raspberries), citrus fruits (like oranges and lemons), kiwi, and papaya. These fruits are rich in vitamin C, a powerful antioxidant that strengthens the immune system and supports overall health.

When it comes to detoxification, cruciferous vegetables like broccoli, cauliflower, kale, and cabbage are particularly noteworthy. These vegetables contain sulfur compounds that aid in the body's detoxification processes, helping to eliminate harmful substances and potentially reducing the risk of cancer.

Understanding the Role of Herbs and Spices in Cancer-Fighting Juices

Herbs and spices not only add flavor to your juices but can also provide additional health benefits. Many herbs and spices have been used for centuries in traditional medicine systems due to their potent medicinal properties.

For example, turmeric contains a compound called curcumin, which has been extensively studied for its anti-inflammatory and anti-cancer effects. Ginger, another popular spice, has been shown to possess antioxidant and anti-inflammatory properties. These herbs and spices can be added to your cancer-fighting juices to enhance their nutritional value and provide potential therapeutic benefits.

Other herbs and spices, such as parsley, cilantro, basil, and mint, not only add freshness and aroma to your juices but also provide additional nutrients and antioxidants. Experimenting with different combinations of herbs and spices can add depth and complexity to your juicing recipes while offering potential health benefits.

Incorporating a wide variety of fruits, vegetables, herbs, and spices into your juicing routine can maximize the nutritional content of your juices and enhance their potential cancer-fighting properties. As you explore the world of juicing, don't be afraid to experiment with different combinations and flavors to find the ones that suit your taste preferences and nutritional needs.

Chapter 3

10 Energizing Breakfast Juices for a Healthy Start

Here are ten juice recipes for energizing breakfasts that can be beneficial for individuals with cancer:

Recipe 1: Carrot-Orange-Ginger Boost

Ingredients:

- 4 carrots
- 2 oranges
- 1-inch piece of ginger

Preparation:

1. Wash and peel the carrots, then cut them into smaller pieces.

2. Peel the oranges and separate them into segments.

3. Peel the ginger and slice it into thin pieces.

4. Put all the ingredients through a juicer.

5. Stir well and enjoy the energizing carrot-orange-ginger boost.

Recipe 2: Green Apple-Celery-Cucumber Refresher

Ingredients:

- 2 green apples

- 2 celery stalks

- 1 cucumber

Preparation:

1. Core the green apples and cut them into chunks.

2. Wash the celery stalks and cucumber, and chop them into smaller pieces.

3. Pass all the ingredients through a juicer.

4. Mix well and savor the refreshing and revitalizing green apple-celery-cucumber refresher.

Recipe 3: Beetroot-Berry Sunrise

Ingredients:

- 1 medium beetroot

- 1 cup mixed of mixed berries (like strawberries, blueberries, raspberries)

- 1 apple

- Juice of 1 lemon

Preparation:

1. Peel and chop the beetroot into smaller pieces.

2. Wash the berries thoroughly.

3. Core the apple and cut it into chunks.

4. Put all the ingredients through a juicer.

5. Stir well and enjoy the vibrant and antioxidant-rich beetroot-berry sunrise juice.

Recipe 4: Spinach-Pineapple-Coconut Delight

Ingredients:

- 2 cups spinach leaves

- 1 cup pineapple chunks

- 1 cup coconut water

- 1 tablespoon chia seeds (optional)

Preparation:

1. Wash the spinach leaves.

2. Juice the spinach and pineapple together.

3. Add the coconut water and chia seeds (if using) to the juice.

4. Mix well and let it sit for a few minutes to allow the chia seeds to swell.

5. Stir again and savor the refreshing and nutrient-packed spinach-pineapple-coconut delight.

Recipe 5: Turmeric-Orange-Carrot Glow

Ingredients:

- 2 oranges

- 2 carrots

- 1-inch piece of turmeric root

- 1 tablespoon honey (optional)

Preparation: Put all the ingredients through a juicer.

1. Peel the oranges and separate them into segments.

2. Wash and peel the carrots, then cut them into smaller pieces.

3. Peel the turmeric root and slice it into thin pieces.

4. Put all the ingredients through a juicer..

5. Add honey if desired for sweetness.

6. Mix well and enjoy the immune-boosting turmeric-orange-carrot glow juice.

Recipe 6: Green Kale-Berry Blast

Ingredients:

- 2 cups kale leaves

- 1 cup of mixed berries (like strawberries, blueberries, raspberries)

- 1 green apple

- Juice of 1 lemon

Preparation:

1. Wash the kale leaves and berries thoroughly.

2. Core the green apple and cut it into chunks.

3. Juice the kale, berries, and apple together.

4. Squeeze the juice of one lemon into the mixture.

5. Stir well and enjoy the antioxidant-rich and nutrient-packed green kale-berry blast.

Recipe 7: Mango-Spinach Smoothie

Ingredients:

- 1 ripe mango

- 2 cups spinach leaves

- 1 cup almond milk

- 1 tablespoon almond butter

- 1 teaspoon honey (optional)

Preparation:

1. Peel and chop the mango.

2. Wash the spinach leaves.

3. Place the mango, spinach, almond milk, almond butter, and honey (if desired) in a blender.

4. Blend until smooth and creamy.

5. Pour into a glass and savor the tropical and nutritious mango-spinach smoothie.

Recipe 8: Blueberry-Banana Oatmeal Smoothie

Ingredients:

- 1 cup blueberries

- 1 ripe banana

- 1 cup almond milk

- ¼ cup rolled oats

- 1 tablespoon flaxseeds

Preparation:

1. Wash the blueberries.

2. Peel and slice the banana.

3. Place the blueberries, banana, almond milk, rolled oats, and flaxseeds in a blender.

4. Blend until smooth and creamy.

5. Pour into a glass and enjoy the nourishing and filling blueberry-banana oatmeal smoothie.

Recipe 9: Watermelon-Strawberry Refresher

Ingredients:

- 2 cups watermelon cubes

- 1 cup strawberries

- Juice of 1 lime

- Mint leaves for garnish

Preparation:

1. Remove the seeds from the watermelon cubes.

2. Wash the strawberries and remove the stems.

3. Place the watermelon cubes and strawberries in

blender.

4. Squeeze the juice of one lime into the blender.

5. Blend until smooth.

6. Pour into a glass, garnish with mint leaves, and enjoy the hydrating and refreshing watermelon-strawberry refresher.

Recipe 10: Papaya-Coconut Paradise

Ingredients:

- 1 ripe papaya

- 1 cup coconut water

- Juice of 1 lime

- Ice cubes (optional)

Preparation:

1. Peel and remove the seeds from the papaya, then cut it into chunks.

2. Place the papaya chunks, coconut water, and lime juice in a blender.

3. Blend until smooth and creamy.

4. Add ice cubes if desired for a chilled beverage.

5. Pour into a glass and savor the tropical and rejuvenating papaya-coconut paradise.

Chapter 4

10 Refreshing Green Juices Packed with Vital Nutrients

Here are ten juice recipes for refreshing green juices packed with vital nutrients that can be beneficial for individuals with cancer:

Recipe 1: Classic Green Detox

Ingredients:

- 2 cups spinach
- 1 cucumber
- 2 celery stalks
- 1 green apple
- Juice of 1 lemon

Preparation:

1. Wash the spinach, cucumber, celery, and green apple.

2. Core the apple and cut it into chunks.

3. Chop the cucumber and celery into smaller pieces.

4. Pass all the ingredients through a juicer.

4. Squeeze the juice of one lemon into the mixture.

5. Mix well and enjoy the refreshing and nutrient-packed classic green detox juice.

Recipe 2: Kale-Pineapple-Mint Delight

Ingredients:

- 2 cups kale leaves

- 1 cup pineapple chunks

- 1 handful of fresh mint leaves

- 1 green apple

Preparation:

1. Wash the kale leaves thoroughly.

2. Core the apple and chop it into chunks.

3. Juice the kale, pineapple, mint leaves, and apple together.

4. Stir well and savor the invigorating and refreshing kale-pineapple-mint delight.

Recipe 3: Cucumber-Spinach-Lime Splash

Ingredients:

- 2 cucumbers

- 2 cups spinach leaves

- Juice of 2 limes

- 1 teaspoon honey (optional)

- Ice cubes (optional)

Preparation:

1. Wash the cucumbers and spinach leaves.

2. Slice the cucumbers into smaller pieces.

3. Juice the cucumbers, spinach leaves, and limes together.

4. Add honey if desired for sweetness.

5. Stir well and pour over ice cubes for a refreshing and hydrating cucumber-spinach-lime splash.

Recipe 4: Green Apple-Celery-Cucumber Cooler

Ingredients:

- 2 green apples

- 4 celery stalks

- 1 cucumber

- Juice of 1 lemon

- A handful of fresh parsley

Preparation:

1. Core the green apples and cut them into chunks.

2. Wash the celery stalks, cucumber, and parsley.

3. Chop the celery and cucumber into smaller pieces.

4. Juice the green apples, celery, cucumber, and parsley together.

5. Squeeze the juice of one lemon into the mixture.

6. Mix well and enjoy the refreshing and nutrient-packed green apple-celery-cucumber cooler.

Recipe 5: Spinach-Kiwi-Cucumber Refresher

Ingredients:

- 2 cups spinach leaves

- 2 kiwis

- 1 cucumber

- Juice of 1 lime

- A handful of fresh mint leaves

Preparation:

1. Wash the spinach leaves, kiwis, cucumber, and minutes leaves.

2. Peel the kiwis and cut them into chunks.

3. Chop the cucumber into smaller pieces.

4. Juice the spinach, kiwis, cucumber, and mint leaves together.

5. Squeeze the juice of one lime into the mixture.

6. Stir well and savor the refreshing and rejuvenating spinach-kiwi-cucumber refresher.

Recipe 6: Green Goddess Smoothie

Ingredients:

- 2 cups kale leaves

- 1 ripe avocado

- 1 banana

- 1 cup almond milk

- 1 tablespoon almond butter

Preparation:

1. Wash the kale leaves.

2. Peel and pit the avocado.

3. Peel the banana.

4. Place the kale, avocado, banana, almond milk, and almond butter in a blender.

5. Blend until smooth and creamy.

6. Pour into a glass and enjoy the nutrient-packed and creamy green goddess smoothie.

Recipe 7: Parsley-Carrot-Apple Elixir

Ingredients:

- 1 bunch of fresh parsley

- 4 carrots

- 2 green apples

- Juice of 1 lemon

Preparation:

1. Wash the parsley and carrots.

2. Chop the parsley and cut the carrots into smaller pieces.

3. Core the green apples and chop them into chunks.

4. Juice the parsley, carrots, and green apples together.

5. Squeeze the juice of one lemon into the mixture.

6. Stir well and savor the revitalizing and nutrient-rich parsley-carrot-apple elixir.

Recipe 8: Green Spinach-Pear Zing

Ingredients:

- 2 cups spinach leaves

- 2 pears

- 1 cucumber

- Juice of 1 lime

- A pinch of cayenne pepper

Preparation:

1. Wash the spinach leaves, pears, and cucumber.

2. Core the pears and cut them into chunks.

3. Chop the cucumber into smaller pieces.

4. Juice the spinach, pears, and cucumber together.

5. Squeeze the juice of one lime into the mixture.

6. Add a pinch of cayenne pepper for an extra kick.

7. Stir well and enjoy the refreshing and zesty spinach-pear zing.

Recipe 9: Green Pineapple-Kale Twist

Ingredients:

- 2 cups kale leaves

- 1 cup pineapple chunks

- 1 green apple

- Juice of 1 lemon

- A handful of fresh cilantro

Preparation:

1. Wash the kale leaves and cilantro.

2. Core the green apple and cut it into chunks.

3. Juice the kale, pineapple, apple, and cilantro together.

4. Squeeze the juice of one lemon into the mixture.

5. Stir well and savor the tangy and revitalizing pineapple-kale twist.

Recipe 10: Minty-Green Melon Splash

Ingredients:

- 2 cups honeydew melon cubes

- 2 cups spinach leaves

- A handful of fresh mint leaves

- Juice of 1 lime

- Ice cubes (optional)

Preparation:

1. Wash the honeydew melon, spinach leaves, and mint leaves.

2. Chop the honeydew melon into smaller cubes.

3. Juice the honeydew melon, spinach leaves, and mint leaves together.

4. Squeeze the juice of one lime into the mixture.

5. Stir well and pour over ice cubes for a refreshing and cooling minty-green melon splash.

Remember, these recipes are intended to supplement a healthy diet and should not replace any medical treatments or advice. It's always a good idea to consult with a healthcare professional before making significant changes to your diet, especially if you're undergoing cancer treatment or have specific dietary restrictions.

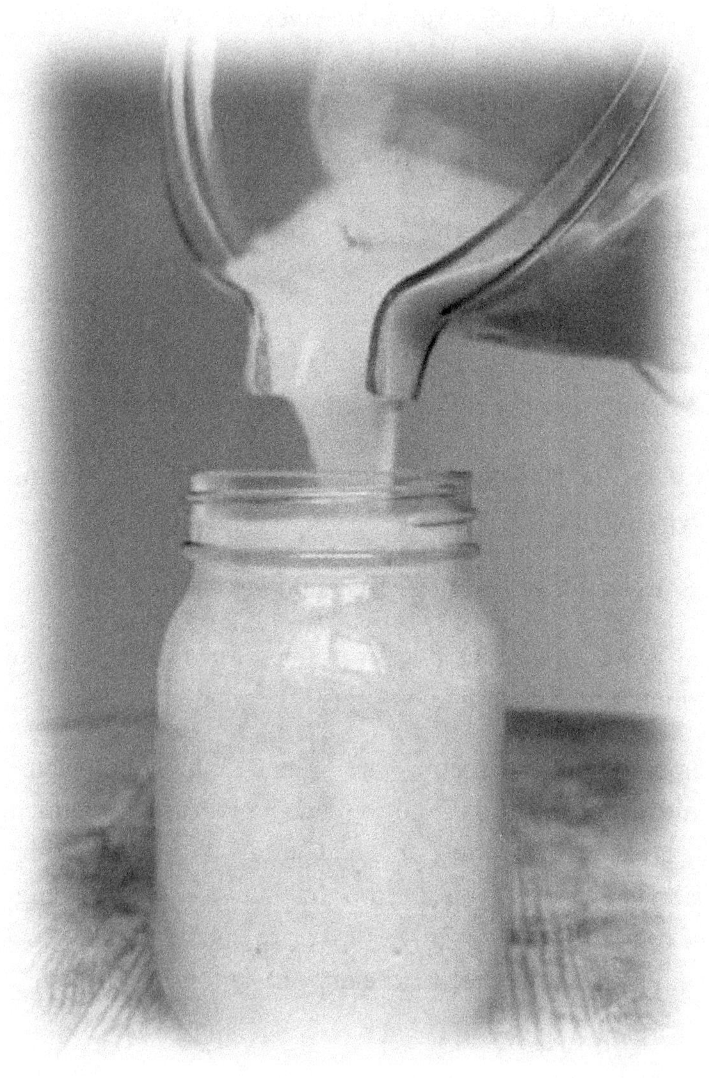

Chapter 5

10 Immunity-Boosting Juices to Enhance Your Defense Mechanisms

Here are ten juice recipes for immunity-boosting juices that can enhance defense mechanisms in individuals with cancer:

Recipe 1: Citrus-Beet Blast

Ingredients:

- 2 oranges
- 1 grapefruit
- 1 small beetroot
- 1-inch piece of ginger

Preparation:

1. Peel the oranges and grapefruit, and separate them into segments.

2. Wash and peel the beetroot, then cut it into smaller pieces.

3. Peel the ginger and slice it into thin pieces.

4. Pass all the ingredients through a juicer.

5. Stir well and enjoy the vibrant and immune-boosting citrus-beet blast.

Recipe 2: Carrot-Turmeric Elixir

Ingredients:

- 4 carrots

- 1 apple

- 1-inch piece of turmeric root

- 1 lemon

Preparation:

1. Wash and peel the carrots, then cut them into smaller pieces.

2. Core the apple and chop it into chunks.

3. Peel the turmeric root and slice it into thin pieces.

4. Juice the carrots, apple, turmeric, and lemon together.

5. Stir well and savor the immune-boosting carrot-turmeric elixir.

Recipe 3: Green Kiwi-Ginger Boost

Ingredients:

- 2 kiwis

- 2 cups spinach leaves

- 1 cucumber

- 1-inch piece of ginger

Preparation:

1. Wash the kiwis, spinach leaves, and cucumber.

2. Peel the kiwis and cut them into chunks.

3. Chop the cucumber into smaller pieces.

4. Peel the ginger and slice it into thin pieces.

5. Pass all the ingredients through a juicer.

6. Mix well and enjoy the refreshing and immunity-enhancing green kiwi-ginger boost.

Recipe 4: Pineapple-Turmeric Twist

Ingredients:

- 2 cups pineapple chunks

- 1 small beetroot

- 1-inch piece of turmeric root

- Juice of 1 lime

Preparation:

1. Wash and peel the beetroot, then cut it into smaller pieces.

2. Peel the turmeric root and slice it into thin pieces.

3. Juice the pineapple, beetroot, turmeric, and lime together.

4. Stir well and savor the tangy and immune-boosting pineapple-turmeric twist.

Recipe 5: Orange-Carrot-Ginger Zinger

Ingredients:

- 4 oranges
- 4 carrots
- 1-inch piece of ginger

Preparation:

1. Peel the oranges and separate them into segments.

2. Wash and peel the carrots, then cut them into smaller pieces.

3. Peel the ginger and slice it into thin pieces.

4. Pass all the ingredients through a juicer.

5. Stir well and enjoy the zesty and immune-boosting orange-carrot-ginger zinger.

Recipe 6: Berry-Antioxidant Powerhouse

Ingredients:

- 1 cup blueberries

- 1 cup strawberries

- 1 cup raspberries

- 1 cup pomegranate seeds

- Juice of 1 lemon

Preparation:

1. Wash the blueberries, strawberries, and raspberries.

2. Remove the stems from the strawberries.

3. Juice the blueberries, strawberries, raspberries, and pomegranate seeds together.

4. Squeeze the juice of one lemon into the mixture.

5. Stir well and savor the antioxidant-rich and immune-boosting berry powerhouse juice.

Recipe 7: Spinach-Orange-Bell Pepper Boost

Ingredients:

- 2 cups spinach leaves

- 2 oranges

- 1 yellow bell pepper

- 1-inch piece of ginger

Preparation:

1. Wash the spinach leaves and bell pepper.

2. Peel the oranges and separate them into segments.

3. Chop the bell pepper into smaller pieces.

4. Peel the ginger and slice it into thin pieces.

5. Pass all the ingredients through a juicer.

6. Mix well and enjoy the invigorating and immune-boosting spinach-orange-bell pepper boost.

Recipe 8: Green Apple-Cucumber-Mint Refresher

Ingredients:

- 2 green apples

- 1 cucumber

- Juice of 1 lemon

- A handful of fresh mint leaves

Preparation:

1. Wash the green apples, cucumber, and mint leaves.

2. Core the apples and chop them into chunks.

3. Chop the cucumber into smaller pieces.

4. Juice the green apples, cucumber, and mint leaves together.

5. Squeeze the juice of one lemon into the mixture.

6. Stir well and enjoy the refreshing and immune-boosting green apple-cucumber-mint refresher.

Recipe 9: Watermelon-Ginger Hydrator

Ingredients:

- 4 cups watermelon cubes

- 1-inch piece of ginger

- Juice of 1 lime

Preparation:

1. Remove the seeds from the watermelon cubes.

2. Peel the ginger and slice it into thin pieces.

3. Juice the watermelon cubes and ginger together.

4. Squeeze the juice of one lime into the mixture.

5. Stir well and savor the hydrating and immune-boosting watermelon-ginger hydrator.

Recipe 10: Tomato-Basil Immune Elixir

Ingredients:

- 4 tomatoes

- 1 cup basil leaves

- Juice of 1 lemon

- A pinch of sea salt

Preparation:

1. Wash the tomatoes and basil leaves.

2. Chop the tomatoes into smaller pieces.

3. Juice the tomatoes and basil leaves together.

4. Squeeze the juice of one lemon into the mixture.

5. Add a pinch of sea salt for taste.

6. Stir well and enjoy the immune-boosting and flavorful tomato-basil elixir.

Remember, these recipes are intended to supplement a healthy diet and should not replace any medical treatments or advice. It's always a good idea to consult with a healthcare professional before making significant changes to your diet, especially if you're undergoing cancer treatment or have specific dietary restrictions.

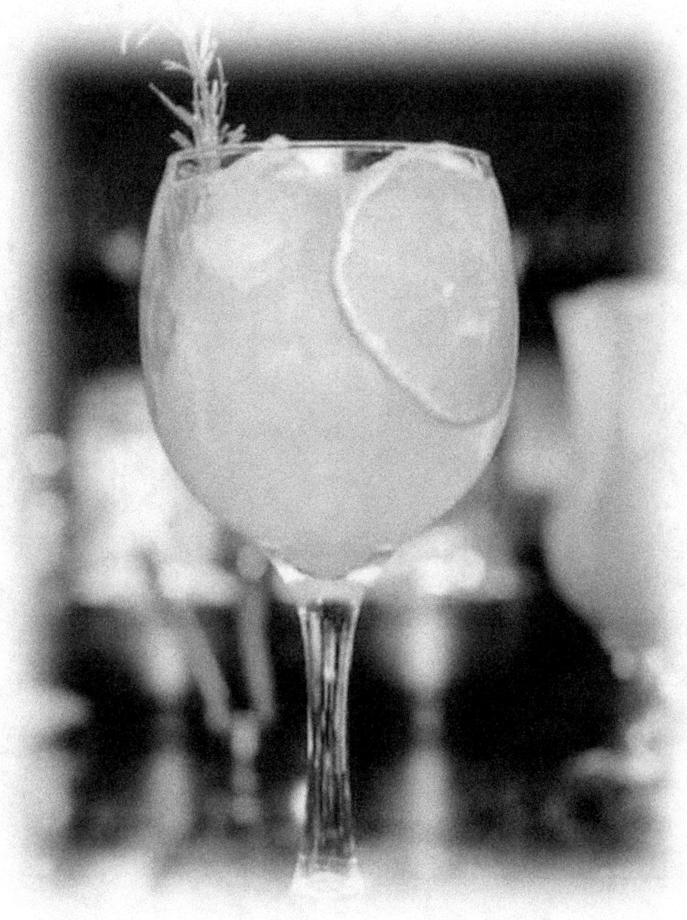

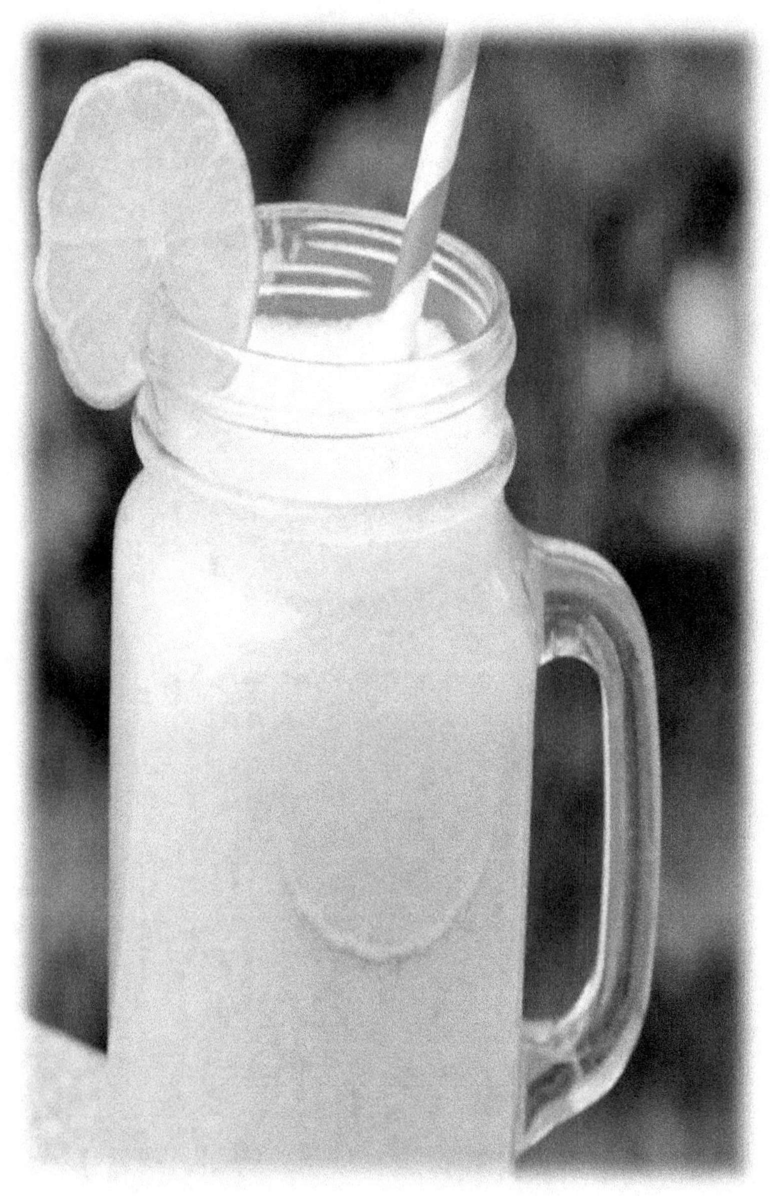

Chapter 6

10 Cleansing and Detoxifying Juices to Support Healing

Here are ten juice recipes for cleansing and detoxifying juices to support healing in individuals with cancer:

Recipe 1: Green Detox Cleanser

Ingredients:

- 2 cups spinach

- 1 cucumber

- 2 celery stalks

- 1 green apple

- 1 lemon

Preparation:

1. Wash the spinach, cucumber, celery, and green apple.

2. Core the apple and cut it into chunks.

3. Chop the cucumber and celery into smaller pieces.

4. Put all the ingredients through a juicer.

5. Squeeze the juice of one lemon into the mixture.

6. Mix well and enjoy the cleansing and detoxifying green detox cleanser.

Recipe 2: Beetroot-Carrot Cleansing Juice

Ingredients:

- 2 beetroots

- 4 carrots

- 1 lemon

- A handful of fresh mint leaves

Preparation:

1. Wash and peel the beetroots and carrots.

2. Chop the beetroots and carrots into smaller pieces.

3. Pass them through a juicer.

4. Squeeze the juice of one lemon into the mixture.

5. Add the fresh mint leaves.

6. Stir well and savor the cleansing and detoxifying beetroot-carrot juice.

Recipe 3: Pineapple-Cucumber-Mint Detox

Ingredients:

- 2 cups pineapple chunks

- 1 cucumber

- Juice of 1 lime

- A handful of fresh mint leaves

Preparation:

1. Wash the pineapple, cucumber, and mint leaves.

2. Chop the pineapple into smaller chunks.

3. Chop the cucumber into smaller pieces.

4. Pass the pineapple and cucumber through a juicer.

5. Squeeze the juice of one lime into the mixture.

6. Add the fresh mint leaves.

7. Stir well and enjoy the refreshing and detoxifying pineapple-cucumber-mint detox juice.

Recipe 4: Lemon-Ginger Cleanse

Ingredients:

- Juice of 2 lemons

- 1 tablespoon grated ginger

- 1 teaspoon raw honey (optional)

- 2 cups filtered water

Preparation:

1. In a glass, squeeze the juice of two lemons..

2. Grate the ginger and add it to the lemon juice.

3. Add raw honey if desired for sweetness.

4. Pour in filtered water and stir well.

5. Let the flavors infuse for a few minutes.

6. Enjoy the cleansing and rejuvenating lemon-ginger cleanse.

Recipe 5: Turmeric-Grapefruit Detoxifier

Ingredients:

- Juice of 2 grapefruits

- 1-inch piece of turmeric root

- A pinch of black pepper

- 2 cups filtered water

Preparation:

1. Squeeze the juice of two grapefruits into a glass.

2. Peel the turmeric root and grate it.

3. Add the grated turmeric and a pinch of black pepper to the grapefruit juice.

4. Pour in filtered water and stir well.

5. Let the flavors infuse for a few minutes.

6. Enjoy the detoxifying and anti-inflammatory turmeric-grapefruit detoxifier.

Recipe 6: Green Kale-Celery Detox Blend

Ingredients:

- 2 cups kale leaves
- 4 celery stalks
- 1 green apple
- 1 cucumber
- Juice of 1 lemon

Preparation:

1. Wash the kale leaves, celery, apple, and cucumber.

2. Core the apple and cut it into chunks.

3. Chop the celery and cucumber into smaller pieces.

4. Juice all of the ingredients in a juicer.

5. Squeeze the juice of one lemon into the mixture.

6. Mix well and enjoy the cleansing and detoxifying green kale-celery detox blend.

Recipe 7: Carrot-Beet Detox Elixir

Ingredients:

- 4 carrots

- 2 beetroots

- 1 lemon

- A handful of fresh cilantro

Preparation:

1. Wash and peel the carrots and beetroots.

2. Chop the carrots and beetroots into smaller pieces.

3. Pass them through a juicer.

4. Squeeze the juice of one lemon into the mixture.

5. Add the fresh cilantro leaves.

6. Stir well and savor the cleansing and detoxifying carrot-beet elixir.

Recipe 8: Watermelon-Mint Detox Refresher

Ingredients:

- 4 cups watermelon cubes

- Juice of 1 lime

- A handful of fresh mint leaves

Preparation:

1. Remove the seeds from the watermelon cubes.

2. Wash the mint leaves.

3. Pass the watermelon cubes through a juicer.

4. Squeeze the juice of one lime into the mixture.

5. Add the fresh mint leaves.

6. Stir well and enjoy the refreshing and detoxifying watermelon-mint detox refresher.

Recipe 9: Cucumber-Lemon-Ginger Detox Splash

Ingredients:

- 1 cucumber

- Juice of 2 lemons

- 1-inch piece of ginger

- A pinch of cayenne pepper

- 2 cups filtered water

Preparation:

1. Wash the cucumber and lemon.

2. Chop the cucumber into smaller pieces.

3. Squeeze the juice of two lemons into a glass.

4. Grate the ginger and add it to the lemon juice.

5. Add a pinch of cayenne pepper.

6. Pour in filtered water and stir well.

7. Let the flavors infuse for a few minutes.

8. Enjoy the cleansing and invigorating cucumber-lemon-ginger detox splash.

Recipe 10: Green Apple-Spinach Detoxifier

Ingredients:

- 2 green apples

- 2 cups spinach leaves

- Juice of 1 lime

- 1 teaspoon spirulina powder (optional)

- 2 cups filtered water

Preparation:

1. Wash the green apples and spinach leaves.

2. Core the apples and cut them into chunks.

3. Pass the apples and spinach through a juicer.

4. Squeeze the juice of one lime into the mixture.

5. Add spirulina powder if desired for an extra detoxifying boost.

6. Pour in filtered water and stir well.

7. Let the flavors infuse for a few minutes.

8. Enjoy the cleansing and nourishing green apple-spinach detoxifier.

Remember, these recipes are intended to supplement a healthy diet and should not replace any medical treatments or advice. It's always a good idea to consult with a healthcare professional before making significant changes to your diet, especially if you're undergoing cancer treatment or have specific dietary restrictions.

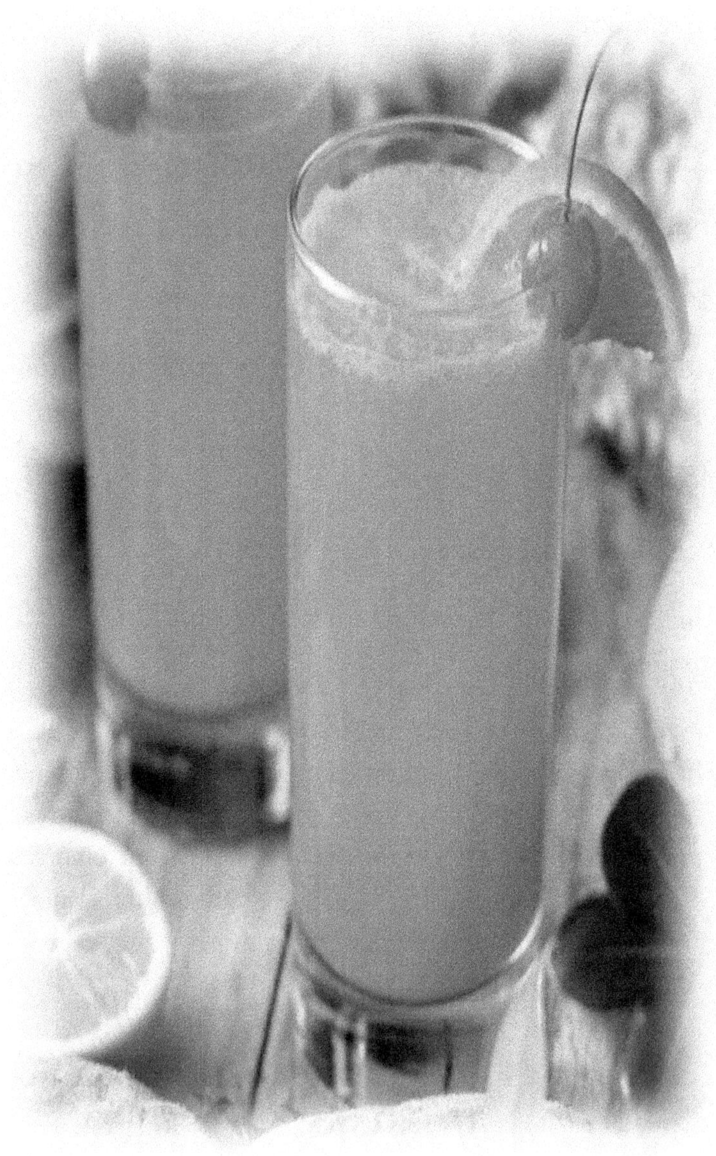

Chapter 7

10 Soothing and Nourishing Juices for Overall Well-being

Here are ten juice recipes for soothing and nourishing juices that promote overall well-being in individuals with cancer:

Recipe 1: Carrot-Orange-Ginger Soother

Ingredients:

- 4 carrots
- 2 oranges
- 1-inch piece of ginger

Preparation:

1. Wash and peel the carrots and oranges.

2. Chop the carrots into smaller pieces.

3. Separate the oranges into segments.

4. Peel the ginger and slice it into thin pieces.

5. Pass all the ingredients through a juicer.

6. Stir well and enjoy the soothing and nourishing carrot-orange-ginger soother.

Recipe 2: Pineapple-Coconut Bliss

Ingredients:

- 2 cups pineapple chunks

- 1 cup coconut water

- 1 banana

- 1 tablespoon chia seeds (optional)

Preparation:

1. Wash and chop the pineapple into smaller chunks.

2. Peel and cut the banana into pieces.

3. Pass the pineapple and banana through a juicer.

4. Pour in the coconut water and stir well.

5. Add chia seeds if desired for an extra nutritional boost.

6. Mix well and savor the tropical and nourishing pineapple-coconut bliss.

Recipe 3: Blueberry-Almond Delight

Ingredients:

- 1 cup blueberries

- 2 cups almond milk

- 1 tablespoon almond butter

- 1 tablespoon honey (optional)

Preparation:

1. Wash the blueberries.

2. Blend the blueberries, almond milk, almond butter, and honey (if using) in a blender until smooth.

3. Pour the mixture into a glass.

4. Stir well and enjoy the creamy and nourishing blueberry-almond delight.

Recipe 4: Spinach-Banana-Pear Soother

Ingredients:

- 2 cups spinach leaves

- 2 bananas

- 2 pears

- Juice of 1 lemon

Preparation:

1. Wash the spinach leaves and pears.

2. Peel the bananas and cut them into slices.

3. Core the pears and chop them into chunks.

4. All of the ingredients should be juiced..

5. Squeeze the juice of one lemon into the mixture.

6. Stir well and savor the soothing and nourishing spinach-banana-pear soother.

Recipe 5: Mango-Coconut-Mint Refresher

Ingredients:

- 2 ripe mangoes

- 1 cup coconut milk

- A handful of fresh mint leaves

- Juice of 1 lime

Preparation:

1. Mangoes should be peeled and cut into bits.

2. Wash the mint leaves.

3. Blend the mangoes, coconut milk, mint leaves, and lime juice in a blender until smooth.

4. Pour the mixture into a glass.

5. Stir well and enjoy the refreshing and nourishing mango-coconut-mint refresher.

Recipe 6: Avocado-Kale Creamy Delight

Ingredients:

- 1 ripe avocado

- 2 cups kale leaves

- 1 green apple

- Juice of 1 lemon

Preparation:

1. Wash the kale leaves and apple.

2. Core the apple and cut it into chunks.

3. Scoop out the avocado flesh.

4. Pass the kale leaves, apple, and avocado through a juicer.

5. Squeeze the juice of one lemon into the mixture.

6. Stir well and savor the creamy and nourishing avocado-kale delight.

Recipe 7: Papaya-Ginger Soother

Ingredients:

- 1 ripe papaya

- 1-inch piece of ginger

- Juice of 1 lime

- 2 cups filtered water

Preparation:

1. Peel and chop the papaya into chunks.

2. Peel the ginger and slice it into thin pieces.

3. Blend the papaya, ginger, lime juice, and filtered water in a blender until smooth.

4. Pour the mixture into a glass.

Stir well and enjoy the soothing and nourishing papaya-ginger soother.

Recipe 8: Raspberry-Coconut Bliss

Ingredients:

- 1 cup raspberries

- 1 cup coconut milk

- 1 tablespoon coconut flakes

- 1 tablespoon honey (optional)

Preparation:

1. Wash the raspberries.

2. Blend the raspberries, coconut milk, coconut flakes, and honey (if using) in a blender until smooth.

3. Pour the mixture into a glass.

4. Stir well and savor the creamy and nourishing raspberry-coconut bliss.

Recipe 9: Turmeric-Apple-Carrot Soother

Ingredients:

- 2 apples

- 2 carrots

- 1-inch piece of turmeric root

- 1 tablespoon honey (optional)

Preparation:

1. Wash and core the apples.

2. Wash and peel the carrots.

3. Peel the turmeric root and slice it into thin pieces.

4. Pass the apples, carrots, and turmeric through a juicer.

5. Add honey if desired for sweetness.

6. Stir well and enjoy the soothing and nourishing turmeric-apple-carrot soother.

Recipe 10: Banana-Oatmeal Energizer

Ingredients:

- 2 bananas

- 1 cup almond milk

- ½ cup cooked oatmeal

- 1 tablespoon almond butter

Preparation:

1. Peel the bananas and cut them into slices.

2. Blend the bananas, almond milk, cooked oatmeal, and almond butter in a blender until smooth.

3. Pour the mixture into a glass.

4. Stir well and enjoy the energizing and nourishing banana-oatmeal energizer.

Remember, these recipes are intended to supplement a healthy diet and should not replace any medical treatments or advice. It's always a good idea to consult with a healthcare professional before making significant changes to your diet, especially if you're undergoing cancer treatment or have specific dietary restrictions.

Chapter 8

5 Juices for Managing Nausea, Fatigue, and Digestive Issues

When dealing with side effects like nausea, fatigue, and digestive issues during cancer treatment, certain juices can help alleviate these symptoms. Here are some juice recipes that may assist in managing these side effects:

1. Ginger-Pear Soother:

Ingredients:

- 1 ripe pear
- 1-inch piece of ginger
- 1 teaspoon lemon juice
- 1 cup coconut water

Preparation:

1. Wash and peel the pear, then cut it into chunks.

2. Peel the ginger and slice it into thin pieces.

3. Combine the pear chunks, ginger, lemon juice, and coconut water in a blender.

4. Blend until smooth.

5. Pour into a glass and sip slowly to soothe nausea and aid digestion.

2. Turmeric-Carrot-Orange Refresher:

Ingredients:

- 2 carrots

- 1 orange

- 1-inch piece of turmeric root

- 1 tablespoon honey (optional)

- 1 cup water

Preparation:

1. Wash and peel the carrots, then chop them into smaller pieces.

2. Peel the orange and separate it into segments.

3. Peel the turmeric root and slice it into thin pieces.

4. Combine the carrot pieces, orange segments, turmeric, honey (if using), and water in a juicer or blender.

5. Blend until well combined.

6. Pour into a glass and consume slowly to reduce inflammation and boost energy levels.

3. Minty Watermelon Cooler:

Ingredients:

- 2 cups watermelon chunks

- 5-6 fresh mint leaves

- Juice of 1 lime

- 1 cup coconut water

Preparation:

1. Wash and chop the watermelon into chunks.

2. Wash the mint leaves.

3. Combine the watermelon chunks, mint leaves, lime juice, and coconut water in a blender.

4. Blend until smooth.

5. Pour into a glass and enjoy this refreshing juice to combat fatigue and stay hydrated.

4. Pineapple-Cucumber Detoxifier:

Ingredients:

- 2 cups pineapple chunks

- 1 cucumber

- 1 teaspoon grated ginger

- Juice of 1 lemon

- 1 cup coconut water

Preparation:

1. Wash and chop the pineapple into chunks.

2. Wash and slice the cucumber.

3. Combine the pineapple chunks, cucumber slices, grated ginger, lemon juice, and coconut water in a blender.

4. Blend until well combined.

5. Pour into a glass and sip slowly to aid digestion and cleanse the body.

5. Papaya-Banana Smoothie:

Ingredients:

- 1 cup ripe papaya chunks

- 1 ripe banana

- 1 cup almond milk

- 1 tablespoon honey (optional)

Preparation:

1. Peel and chop the papaya into chunks.

2. Peel the banana and cut it into slices.

3. Combine the papaya chunks, banana slices, almond milk, and honey (if using) in a blender.

4. Blend until smooth.

5. Pour into a glass and consume slowly to ease digestive issues and provide a nourishing energy boost.

Remember, individual preferences and tolerances may vary, so adjust the ingredients and quantities according to your needs. If you have specific dietary restrictions or concerns, consult with a healthcare professional or registered dietician for personalized advice tailored to your condition.

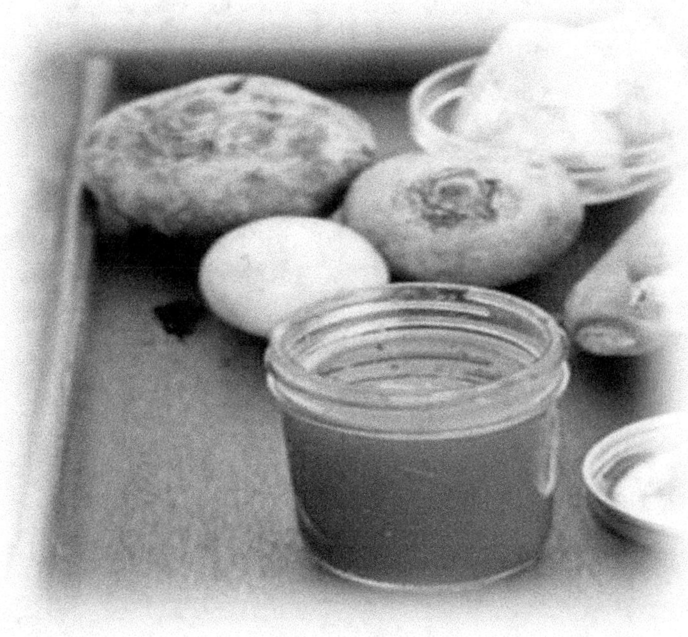

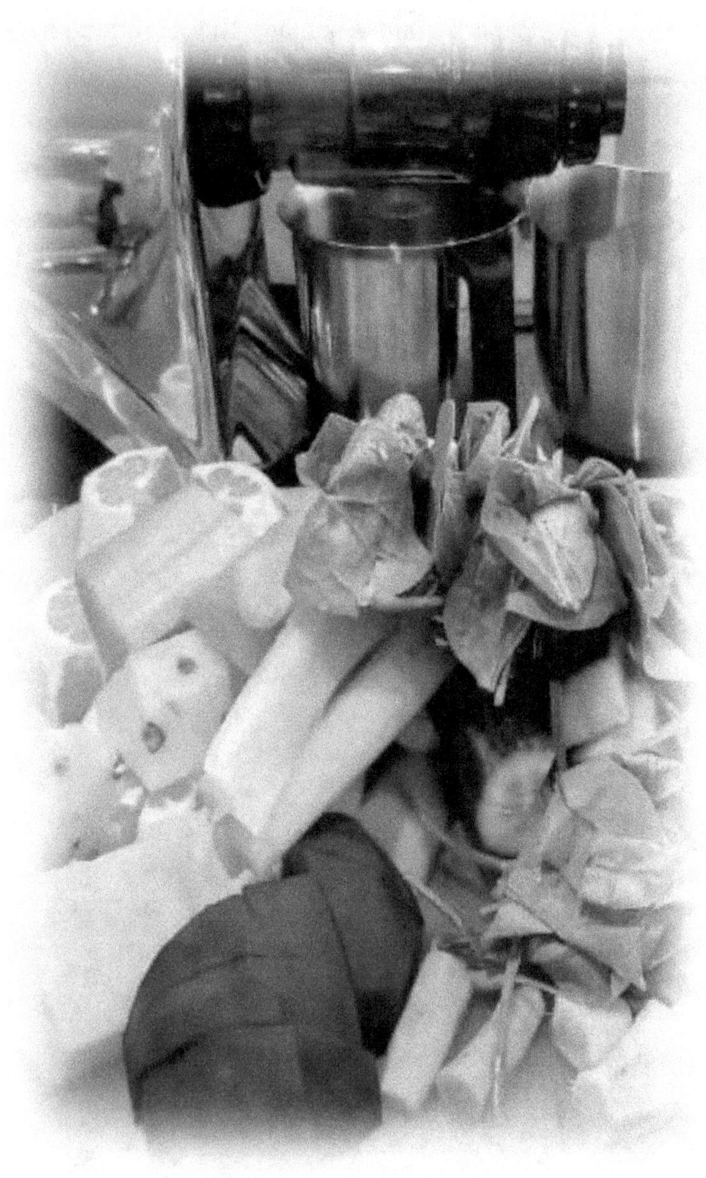

Chapter 9

Timing and Frequency: When and How to Consume Juices

Timing and frequency of consuming juices for individuals with cancer can vary depending on individual preferences, medical conditions, and treatment plans. However, consider the following general guidelines:

1. **Morning:** Many people prefer to start their day with a fresh juice to kickstart their metabolism and provide a boost of nutrients. Consuming a juice in the morning on an empty stomach allows for better absorption of the nutrients. It can also help to hydrate the body after a night's sleep.

2. **Between meals**: Drinking juices between meals can help maintain steady energy levels and provide a nutrient boost. Aim for mid-morning or mid-afternoon to prevent any interference with digestion during mealtime.

3. **Pre-workout:** If you engage in physical activity, consuming a juice before your workout can provide a natural source of energy and hydration. Opt for juices that contain easily digestible carbohydrates for quick energy.

4. **Post-workout:** After exercising, it's important to replenish your body with fluids and nutrients. Juices with a balance of carbohydrates, proteins, and electrolytes can

help in recovery. Consider adding a source of protein like nut milk or protein powder to aid in muscle repair.

5. **Avoiding mealtimes:** It's generally recommended to consume juices away from main meals to prevent dilution of digestive juices and potential interference with the digestion of solid foods. Wait at least 30 minutes before or after a meal to drink juice.

6. **Spread throughout the day:** Instead of consuming large quantities of juice in one sitting, it may be more beneficial to spread the intake throughout the day. This allows for a continuous supply of nutrients and helps prevent a sudden spike in blood sugar levels.

7. **Freshly prepared:** To maximize the nutritional content and freshness of the juices, it's best to prepare them just before consuming. Freshly squeezed or blended juices contain higher levels of enzymes, antioxidants, and other beneficial compounds.

8. **Variety is key:** Incorporate a variety of fruits, vegetables, and herbs into your juices to ensure a wide range of nutrients. Experiment with different combinations and flavors to keep it interesting and to provide a diverse nutrient profile.

9. **Moderation:** While juices can be beneficial, it's important not to over consume them. They should be seen as a supplement to a well-rounded diet, not a replacement for whole foods. Remember to consider the calorie content

of the juices and adjust your overall calorie intake accordingly.

10. **Personalization**: Consult with a healthcare professional, such as a registered dietician or nutritionist, who can provide personalized recommendations based on your specific needs, medical condition, and treatment plan.

Remember that these guidelines are general and may need to be adjusted based on individual circumstances. It's always advisable to consult with a healthcare professional for personalized advice tailored to your specific needs.

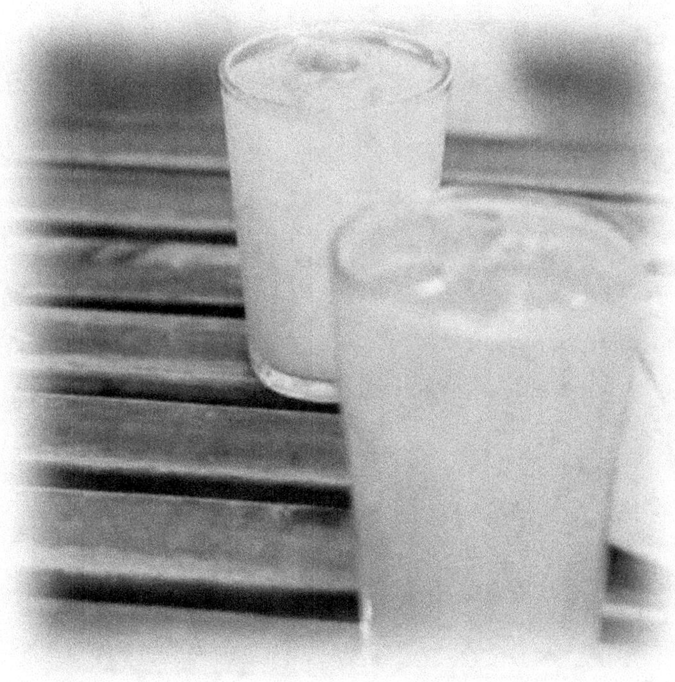

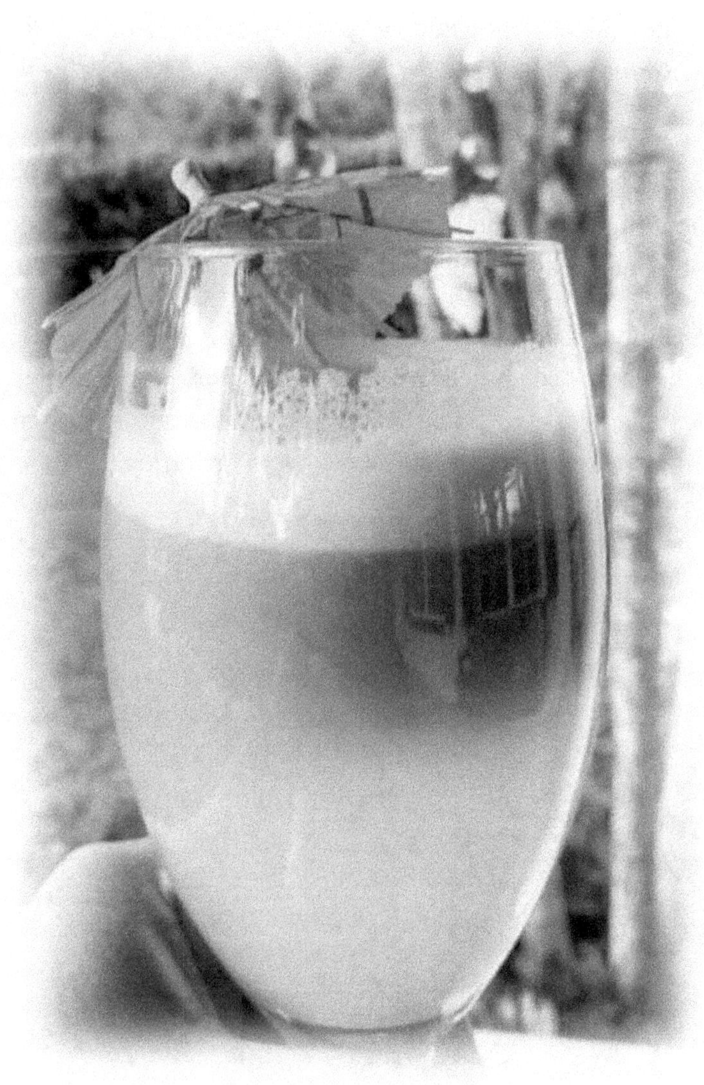

Chapter 10

Frequently Asked Questions about Juicing for
Cancer

Here are answers to frequently asked questions about
juicing for cancer:

Q: Can juicing alone cure cancer?

A: No, juicing alone cannot cure cancer. While juicing can
provide a concentrated source of nutrients and support
overall health, it is not a substitute for medical treatments
such as chemotherapy, radiation, or surgery. Juicing should
be seen as a complementary approach to a comprehensive
cancer treatment plan.

**Q: Are there any side effects of juicing for cancer
patients?**

A: In general, fresh juices made from fruits and vegetables
are safe for most people. However, some individuals may
experience digestive issues such as diarrhea, bloating, or
gas due to the high fiber content in certain juices.
Additionally, some juices may interact with medications or
specific medical conditions. It's important to listen to your
body and consult a healthcare professional if you
experience any adverse effects.

Q: Can juicing interact with cancer medications?

A: Some juices may interact with certain cancer medications. For example, grapefruit juice can interfere with the metabolism of certain drugs, leading to higher levels of the medication in the body. It's important to inform your healthcare provider about any dietary changes, including juicing, to ensure there are no potential interactions with your specific medications.

Q: Should I consult a healthcare professional before starting juicing?

A: Yes, it's highly recommended to consult with a healthcare professional, such as a registered dietician or nutritionist, before starting juicing or making significant dietary changes, especially if you're undergoing cancer treatment or have specific medical conditions. They can provide personalized guidance, take into account your medical history, and ensure that juicing aligns with your overall treatment plan.

Remember, while juicing can be a beneficial addition to a cancer patient's diet, it's important to approach it as part of a comprehensive treatment plan and not rely solely on juicing for cancer management. Individualized guidance from healthcare professionals is crucial for optimal outcomes.

Conclusion

In conclusion, juicing can be a valuable addition to the lives of individuals facing the challenges of cancer. While it is essential to understand that juicing alone cannot cure cancer, it can serve as a powerful tool to enhance overall well-being, support the immune system, and provide a concentrated source of vital nutrients.

Throughout this book, we have explored the foundations of juicing for cancer, delving into the basics of cancer, common types, treatment options, and the role of nutrition in prevention and treatment. We have discovered the benefits of juicing, including its ability to provide a plethora of antioxidants, phytochemicals, and essential vitamins and minerals that can support the body's natural defense mechanisms.

From energizing breakfast juices to refreshing green blends and immunity-boosting elixirs, we have provided a diverse range of recipes to suit different tastes and nutritional needs. These recipes have been carefully crafted to incorporate a variety of fruits, vegetables, herbs, and spices known for their potential cancer-fighting properties.

It is important to note that while juicing can offer numerous health benefits, it should never replace conventional medical treatments or professional advice. Juicing should always be viewed as a complement to a comprehensive cancer treatment plan, implemented with the guidance of healthcare professionals who can consider individualized needs and potential interactions with medications.

In the journey of cancer, juicing can play a role in managing side effects such as nausea, fatigue, and digestive issues. With recipes tailored to address these symptoms, individuals can find comfort and nourishment during their treatment process.

It is our hope that this book has provided you with valuable insights, inspiration, and practical knowledge to embark on your juicing journey with confidence. We encourage you to explore and experiment with different ingredients, listen to your body's needs, and seek support from healthcare professionals who can guide you on this path.

Remember, the power of juicing lies not only in the physical benefits it may provide but also in the joy, mindfulness, and connection it can foster with our bodies and overall well-being. May your juicing experience be filled with health, healing, and a renewed sense of vitality as you navigate your journey toward wellness.

Wishing you strength, resilience, and abundant health.